Soap Making:

25 Natural Homemade Soap Recipes for Home

Table of content

Introduction

Research suggests that soap was being used as long ago as 2800 B.C. The ancient Babylonians are thought to have made soap from ashes and fat, although it is unknown as to the extent that soap was used by the general population.

There is also evidence to suggest that the Ancient Egyptians, from approximately 1500 B.C. used a soap product created by mixing fatty animal oils with salt; in effect create a soap which would exfoliate as well! Even the Romans are known to have made a form of soap from urine!

Soap is, in effect a vital part of human history, whether washing blood from your hands in ancient times or destroying microscopic germs; it has always been used. Of course, the more modern versions of soap have been created to leave a pleasant aroma as well as effective and gently washing the skin.

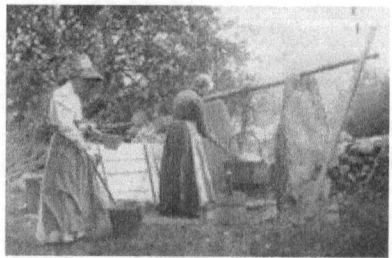

As with most products, soap was originally something that only the richest people could afford; there were very few people capable or licensed to make soap and they guarded their skills carefully. They general used animal oil and parts of plants to create distinctive soaps. This ensured an elite class of customer. However, at the end of the 18th century, a Frenchman discovered a way of chemical making soap; this was the first time soap could be made on a much larger scale. This was the catalyst which drove the price of soap down and made it affordable to a much wider range of people.

This discovery was followed in the early part of the 19th century that soap could be made from glycerin, fats and acid. This made it even cheaper to create soap and is considered to be the foundations of modern soap making; there have been no significant advancements in the science of soap making since. The techniques and principles which were first used approximately two hundred years ago, are still in use today!

Of course, modern technology has changed the understanding of soap, he ingredients are better understood and broken down which has enabled the creation of different types of soap for different situations. Laundry soap is one example of a product which is subtly different to hand soap or even bathing soaps; each has its own role to fulfill. It was only in the 1970's that liquid soap became possible, it has become exceptionally popular since and helps to promote hand washing as well as minimize soap wastage.

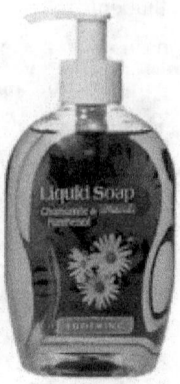

The modern world has a dazzling array if soaps, depending upon your needs, how you wish to smell and even what type of skin you have. These constant changes, improvements and marketing ploys help to keep soap fresh in everyone's mind; a standard bar of soap may be less popular, but the concept and use of soaps has never been so popular. There remains a thriving market for commercially created soaps, there is also a place for those who wish to create their own, homemade soap; a process which I surprisingly easy!

This book will guide you through the best method to make soap and the tools and equipment you will need to complete this task at home. It will also provide you with a selection of twenty five recipes to help you practice and create your own soap; you should then be able to discover and make hundreds of other types of soap!

Chapter 1 – The Need For Soap and How to Make It

In the modern world everyone is aware of the need for soap and its role in helping us to stay clean and healthy, although many people are unaware of how soap works and how regularly it should be used. In fact, there have been many studies into the effects of soap. There are even those who believe that soap is not necessary; the body is able to clean itself. There are two main uses of soap:

Odor Removal

In general research agrees that young children, male or female do not have any odor creating regions. It is, therefore, not necessary for children to use soap in order to remove unpleasant body odors, although soap can still be used to aid them in smelling nice. However, adults, particularly men, do have odor producing regions. Research suggests that it is essential to soap these regions every two days unless you partake in very physical work; in which case every day is essential. Water by itself can significantly reduce the presence if body odor, but will not eliminate it completely. Deodorant will always be needed to assist with reducing and containing odors, the regularity of application will be directly related to the physical duties undertaken. Washing in water will help to reduce body odor but it is more effective when mixed with soap.

Cleanliness

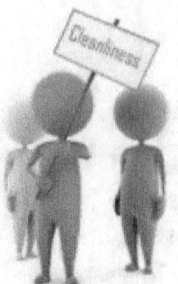

Soap has always been acknowledged as a way to remove dirt and germs from your hands, this is via a process of friction and agitation; in fact, modern soaps have small particles added to them to aid with dirt removal and the removal of excess skin. The abrasive nature of these products will help to leave your skin fresh and glowing and will often help to keep skin conditions at bay. This is because many soap products are becoming more technologically advanced and are able to offer deep pore washes.

There is a school of thought which recommends using only water to clean the skin. However, with the advancements in modern science washing soap can do much more than simple wash your skin, it can help t protect, moisturize and even keep you looking younger for longer.

It is the amount of science behind the soap that often worries people regarding what they are really putting on their face or body. This is one of the main reasons people start to make their own soap; knowing which ingredients have been placed into a bar means you know what you are putting on your body.

The basic process of making any soap is surprisingly simple, in fact, the most important question you will need to ask yourself is whether you wish to handle Lye yourself or not. Lye is a natural product, also known as Sodium Hydroxide. It is an alkali and can be dangerous; it is capable of making a hole in your fabrics and can burn your skin. However, as long as you handle it with care there will be no issue using it; it is worth noting that you should always use the crystal version of Lye when making salt and it must always be added to the water, not the water to it.

This lye, added in the right quantities to plain water can then be mixed with a variety of different oil. The mixture bonds together to create soap; the main difference between recipes is the additional flavorings and the type of oil used. Every oil has its own specific relationship to lye and must be used in the right quantities.

If the thought of handling lye is to daunting for you at first, then you can purchase a melt and pour soap which is ready to use. As its name suggests, you simply melt it, add your own flavors and pour it into the molds.

The basic tools and equipment required are covered in the next chapter.

Chapter 2 – Tools and Equipment

Thankfully most of the items you will need you will already own; they are normal kitchen utensils. It is worth noting that if you intend to create your own soap on a regular basis is could be worth purchasing equipment specifically for your soap making. This will ensure there is no tang of soap left when cooking your evening meal!

Of course, as well as having all the right tools to hand, you will need to have chosen one of the recipes in this book and made sure that you either have the necessary ingredients or that you have acquired. It can be surprisingly cost effective, as well as fun to make your own soap.

Essential Tools;

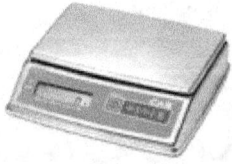

- Scales – the best ones are digital as the more soap you make the more precise you will be regarding the ingredients. This is not just in an effort to reproduce a bar of soap; very small changes in the ingredients can affect the oiliness of the finished product.

- Jars and bowls; these should, ideally, be made of glass.

- Spoons; the best option is to have a wooden one, a metal one and a plastic one.

- Something to contain and shape your soap. You can buy purpose made molds, or you can use a variety of items from your home. Silicon cake tins are one option, but a cardboard box lined with parchment paper can work just as well.

- Gloves are essential as the mixture will be hot, if you decide to use Lye it can also be harmful to your skin. It is also advisable to have some sort of eye protection; this will help prevent splashes from damaging your eyes.

- Vinegar – this will effectively counteract the lye if you do have an accident with it. Having a bottle to hand means you will be ready and able to prevent a disaster!

- A blender; this will make mixing and creating your soap much easier! This should be the handheld, stick type.

- A mixing bowl; the size of this will depend upon the amount of soap you wish to make. For your first attempts it is advisable to make a small amount and get a feel for how to make soap; you will then be able to tweak recipes to suit your own requirements.

- Cloths; you will need to react quickly to any spills; a cloth or paper towel is the best option for this.

You may also wish to consider having a selection of plastic cups handy; this will help you to have the oils and fragrances pre-measured and ready to add to your mix.

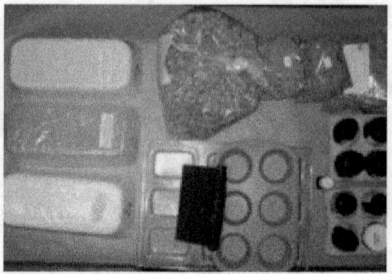

Having got all your tools to hand and your ingredients you will be ready to get started. Perhaps the most important thing to remember when making soap is that preparation is everything. You variety of containers will ensure you are able to measure and prepare all the ingredients before you start mixing them together; doing this will make the process much easier.

Chapter 3 – 10 Fantastic Soaps for All Occasions

There are literally hundreds of potential combinations and types of soap which can be made. In fact, some if the best ones are made as a result of trial and error. The best approach to learning how to make soap is to use the recipes in this book, follow the instructions and understand the process. Once you have mastered this you will be able to change the ingredients and try some of your own combinations, just be sure to note down what you are doing so that you can reproduce it if necessary!

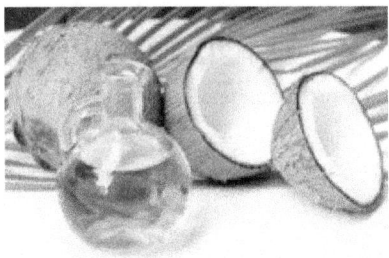

Coconut Oil Soap for Washing

You will need 33 ounces of Coconut Oil, 4.75 ounces of lye and 12.5 ounces of water. If you wish to you can also an a few drops of essential oils.

It is worth noting that there are various types of coconut oil which melt at different temperatures. Ideally you should use one which melts at 76 degrees Fahrenheit, although the recipe will work well with any coconut oil.

The first step is to measure out your three key ingredients. You need to add the water to an empty bowl and then slowly pour the lye into the water. It is advisable to avoid breathing in the fumes whilst doing this. By pouring the lye slowly you will reduced the chance of splash-back and help it to dissolve effectively. The mixture will take approximately ten minutes to go clear.

Separately you will need to put your coconut oil into a pan and heat it to around 120 Fahrenheit. It should melt into a clear liquid.

You can then merge the two liquids carefully together. You can then use your blender to gentle mix it until it appears creamy and light. You can then put the mixture on a low heat and allow to simmer for approximately three quarters of an hour. The soap should be half clear; much like Vaseline. You can check it is ready by making sure it is between seven and ten on a piece of PH paper.

As it cools add your essential oils and then spoon the mixture into your chosen molds. It can cool naturally or cool in the fridge for a quicker result. It is usable straight away although it will be at its best a couple of weeks after production.

Coconut Oil Laundry Soap

This is the same ingredients as the soap for washing but it is important to use one ounce more of lye and half an ounce less of water. The rest of the process is the same but it will make a bar which is more appropriate for washing clothes in.

Olive Oil Soap

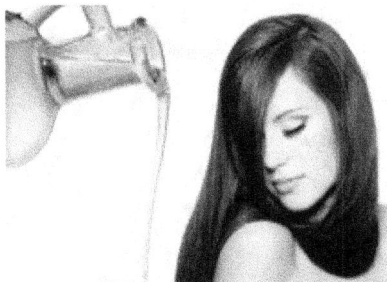

The ingredients in this are very similar to those in coconut oil soap. You will need 50 oz of olive oil, 6.3 oz of Lye and 15 oz of water.

You can choose whether to make the lye first or the olive oil. The water needs to be placed into a good sized bowl or container and the lye slowly added. Again, it will take approximately ten minutes to dissolve completely.

The olive oil will need heating on the stove to ensure it is hot, but not necessarily boiling. You can then slowly add this to the lye mixture and start blending. It should take between five and ten minutes to become nice and creamy.

You will then be able to fill your prepared molds and leave to set. They should, ideally be left overnight and they must be covered to ensure they harden properly.

Poppy seed Soap

Instead of using lye it is possible to use a soap base. This can be bought at most craft shops and will vary in price depending upon what the base is created from.

You will also need poppy seeds and you may wish to use coloring to ensure you soap look good.

Ideally you should use 10 oz of your soap base. Cut it into small pieces and place in a jug or bowl. This can then be melted in the microwave. Once melted add a teaspoon of poppy seeds and a few drops of coloring if required. You can also add a fragrance if desired. Mix all the ingredients and pour into your mold.

Put the mold in the fridge for fifteen minutes and then the soap is ready to us.

Jasmine and Rosewood

You will need one teaspoon of kaolin clay, two teaspoons of titanium dioxide, half an ounce of jasmine and half an ounce of rosewood. You will also need five ounces of lye, twelve ounce of water and possibly yellow oxide.

Start by adding the lye slowly to the water and leaving it to clear, (as before). Then mix the titanium dioxide and clay together; you will need to grind them to ensure there are no lumps. You can then add the jasmine, rosewood and titanium mixture to the lye, stirring carefully whilst doing so. You may also wish to add a little yellow oxide to improve the color of the soap.

Once mixed, you can pour into your chosen molds and leave for twenty four hours before cutting into blocks. It is best to leave the cut soap for three weeks before using it.

Calendula soap

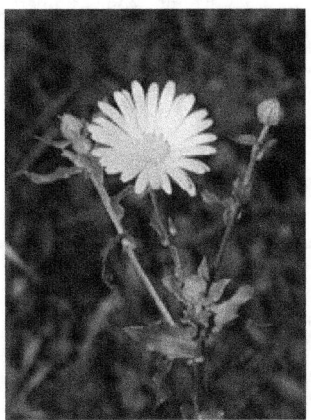

You will need; 21 ounces of olive oil, 14 ounces of coconut oil, 2 ounces of castor oil, 5 ounces of sunflower oil, 13 ounces of calendula tea, 6 ounces of lye and 13 ounces of water.

As usual measure out the water and slowly add the lye to it, then wait for it to become clear. Mix the oils together and heat them until they nearly reach boiling point, the slowly add them to the lye mix. Now simply add the calendula tea and blend until creamy.

You will then be able to pour them into your molds and use your soap in a couple of weeks.

Shampoo bar

As its name suggests this product is perfect for washing your hair! You will need; 9 ounces of olive oil and coconut oil, 4 ounces of coconut oil and of jojoba oil, two ounces of shea butter and cocoa butter, one ounce beeswax, four ounces water and four ounces of lye,

As usual, slowly add the lye to the water. Whilst this is becoming clear, mix all the oils and the beeswax together. This mixture can then be heated, but not brought to the boil. Now mix the lye with the oils and b lend until it is thick and creamy. The mixture should then be allowed to simmer for one hour and then you can pour it into its molds. After twenty four hours the mold can be cut into bar and left to cool further; although they can be used straight away.

Gin and Tonic Soap

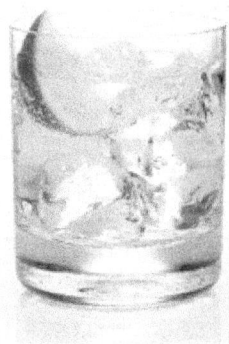

As with all the recipes you will need to pour 5 ounces of lye into 12 ounces of water and allow it to mix to makes its own, clear liquid.

You will then need to heat 3.5 ounces of olive oil, 2.5 ounces coconut oil, 1.5 ounces shea butter, 1.5 ounces lard and 1 ounce of castor oil. Do not allow it to boil before you add it the lye and water. This should then be left for approximately six hours; then add half an ounce of juniper oil, 3 ounces of lemon essential oil and a teaspoon of kaolin clay. Cut after twenty four hours and use after three weeks.

Lanolin Shaving soap

Lanolin is a natural moisturizer and is perfect for shaving with as it prevents the skin from drying out as you shave. To create it you will need the following ingredients:

1 ounce kokum butter, 2 ounces lanolin, 2 ounces of shea butter, 11 ounces of coconut oil, 10 ounces of rice bran oil, 7 ounces palm kernel flakes, 1 ounce

pumpkin oil. You will also need 5 ounces of lye and twelve ounces of water and you can add any essential oil you like to create a pleasant fragrance.

Mix the water and lye as usual, whilst waiting for it to cool and clear you should mix all the other oils and butter together, heat all these ingredients until they are all melted. Ideally you should merge the two liquids at approximately 110 degrees. Just prior to merging you can add the essential oils.

Once merged blend into a cream and then put into your molds. Keep them wrapped and insulated for twenty four hours before cutting them to size. Then keep them stored for another three weeks before using them.

Aloe Vera Soap

As with all these soaps you will need to prepare a mixture of lye and water before mixing the oils whilst heating and then combining the two mixtures. For this recipe you need 10 ounces of lye and 7 ounces of lye.

The oils which need to be mixed are 15 ounces Coconut oil, 13 Ounces olive oil and 10 ounces lard. Just prior to mixing them with the lye, it is essential to add the aloe gel. Once they have been blended it will take about 48 hours for them to be set enough to cut and a further four weeks before they should be used.

Chapter 4 – 10 Food Flavoured Soap

There are a great many number of soaps which have been created using food flavorings; this can add a beautiful fragrance to any soap and can also provide a host of health benefits. The following recipes all use the same approach as the soaps already described. Every soap mixture requires 12 ounces of water and 5 ounces of lye. Your soap making should start by carefully mixing these together. The mixture will go cloudy and become extremely hot. Whilst this is settling you should mix the oils and warm them. Add any essential oils can be added prior to mixing lye and the oils.

The following recipes all adopt this approach, as such, only the ingredients and items which need to be noted will appear:

Honey Soap

Additional ingredients to the lye and water are; one tablespoon of buttermilk fragrance oil, half a tablespoon of vanilla flavoring, orange color, (you can choose not to use this) and 3 ounces of honey. Your choice of honey will affect the color of your soap and hence affect whether you wish to use the orange coloring or not. You may also like to find bee molds or honeycombs to make the soap more fun!

Chai Latte Soap

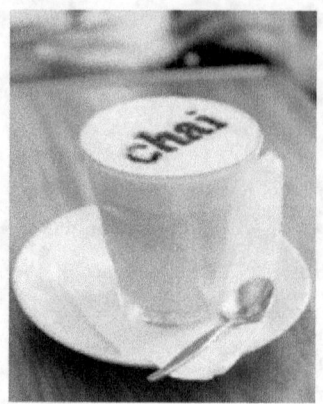

You will need five ounces of coconut oil, five ounces of olive oil and five ounces of olive oil. You will then also need two ounces of cocoa butter and two ounces of castor oil. The ingredients should all be mixed and blended as per the usual instructions. However, you will notice it thickens quickly when blended. It can also look fantastic to make them in plastic cups; you can even decorate the top and make two batches to create the milky layer and the coffee layer; so that they look like a coffee/ latte!

Chocolate Soap

Who wouldn't want to wash in a bar of chocolate! This soap is created to look exactly like a bar of chocolate, or, if stood on its end it could be a hot chocolate!

You will need; four ounces of olive oil, two and a half ounces of coconut oil, two ounces of lard, one ounce of avocado oil and half an ounce of castor oil. You will also need two teaspoons of whole milk powder, two of coffee granules, one teaspoon of cocoa powder and 2 teaspoons of vanilla flecks. Additionally, you will need two teaspoons of red clay and two of brown clay, along with two teaspoons of vanilla flavoring.

The oils should be mixed with the lye as usual; once it has been blended and become creamy you can add the extra ingredients and pour into a mold. As usual the soap can be cut to size within twenty four hours and then left for three weeks to harden

Candy cane Christmas Soap

You will need; 4 ounces of olive oil, 2.5 ounces of coconut oil, 2 ounces of lard, 1 ounce of avocado oil and half an ounce of castor oil. You will also need two teaspoons of peppermint essence, one teaspoon of vanilla essence, one tablespoon kaolin clay, half a teaspoon of red oxide and half a teaspoon of green oxide.

Mix the lye and heat the oils as normal. Then add the vanilla and peppermint essence and blend in the kaolin clay. Now split the soap mix into three bowls.

Add the red oxide to one bowl and the green oxide to another. Now alternate and swirl the colors separately into the molds. They should create a candy cane effect. As usual leave for twenty four hours before cutting and leave for a further thre weeks before using.

Milk Soap

You will need 20 ounces of milk, twenty ounces of coconut oil, four ounces of your preferred fragrance and four pounds of lard. As usual you can start by preparing the lye and water. You will need to wait for approximately an hour for the mixture to lower its temperature to approximately eighty degrees. You can then add the cold milk. Whilst the temperature is settling again you can prepare the oil and the lard; merging them and heating them to ninety degrees. You can then add the oils to the lye and keep stirring until it is thick.

You can then pour it into your chosen molds, but you must cover the mold with plastic and a blanket; this will ensure the heat is retained which will effectively cook the soap. Again, after twenty four hours it can be cut into shapes or the size required. It should be allowed to air dry for another four weeks before being used.

Creamy Orange Soap

This soap requires two tablespoons of annatto seeds, two ounces of olive oil, two tablespoons of poppy seeds, one ounce of essential oil; orange flavored preferably and one and a half ounces of peppermint oil.

Mix the oils heat them with the essential oils and seeds. The simply merge them with the lye mixture and blend. You should then be able to pour the mixture into the mold and leave for twenty four hours to set.

The seeds will act as an exfoliate in the soap making it very good at restoring dry skin.

Marbled Beer Soap

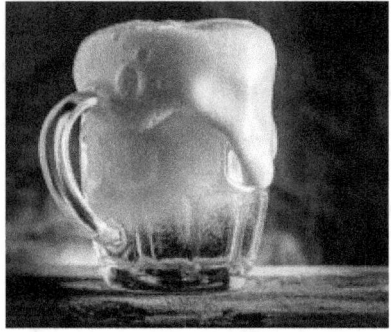

You may not know whether to wash with this or drink it, but it will certainly make a good talking point and a gift. You need four and a half ounces of chilled beer, five ounces of palm kernel oil, three and a half ounces of palm oil and the same of coconut oil. You will also need one ounce of Babassu oil, five ounces of rapeseed oil, five ounces of sunflower oil, one ounce of castor oil, two ounces of soybean oil and half an ounce of cedar wood essential oil.

Having collected all the ingredients together you should introduce half of the lye to the water as normal; the other half should be poured into the cold beer. Heat your oils and merge them with your water and with your beer; roughly half the oils inn each pot. You will not be able to blend this to a thick consistency. Now pour the two mixtures into the mold, you can alternate or even pour at the same time to achieve a marble effect. You can then cover it for between twenty four and forty eight hours, keeping it warm to help it set.

Apple Cider Soap

In this mixture, instead of adding your lye to water, add it to nine ounces of chilled cider. You can then mix your oils; 15 ounces of olive oil, 2 ounces castor oil, 8 ounces coconut oil, 2 ounces cocoa butter and 3 ounces of avocado oil. You can also add a touch of ginger or cinnamon, to your own preference.

Cinnamon Soap

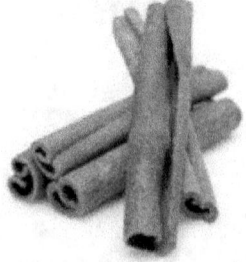

The oil mixture consists of 3.5 ounces olive oil, 2.5 ounces coconut oil, 1.5 ounces lard, 1.5 ounces shea butter and 1 ounce castor oil. You will also need a teaspoon of ground cinnamon, a tablespoon of white clay and two teaspoons of cinnamon essential oil. The essential oil, ground cinnamon and clay should be added at the end of the process; just before you pour the soap into the molds.

Tea Tree Soap

This soap requires an oil mixture of 14 ounces olive oil, 10 ounces coconut oil, 4 ounces sweet almond oil, 4 ounces avocado oil and two teaspoons of tea tree essential oil. Again, the tea tree essential oil should be added just before the soap is poured into the mold. After twenty four hours you can cut the mold and it can be left to air dry for up to six weeks.

Chapter 5 – A selection of fun Soaps – 5 Recipes

The list of soaps you can make is endless; in fact, you are only limited by your imagination. It is even possible to use a soap base instead of the lye to avoid the danger involved in dealing with lye. The following five recipes are done using a soap base but are all worth trying: Each recipe requires you to melt the soap base in the microwave and then add the necessary ingredients to make your soap. Solid particles will go to the bottom of the soap unless you allow it to set a little first.   The soap can set in as little as three hours although it is always recommended to chill it overnight.

Herbs & Citrus Soap

Simply put some soap base in a bowl, or grate an old bar of soap and warm it up. Soap base can be warmed in the microwave whereas old soap is best to do on the stove. Simply choose your favorite hers, such as mint or rosemary and grind or puree them into tiny pieces. Once your base has melted, and them to it and stir in. Pour the soap into the molds and leave to cool for an hour; you can speed the cooling and setting process by putting them in the freezer.

Mocha Soap

Simply melt the soap base and add approximately one tablespoon of coffee and cocoa powder to it. This will create a fantastic smelling soap. To help create the mocha effect you could melt a second soap base and add a little white colorant to help create the milky mocha effect. To make a stunning display pour the two soap bases into a cup at the same time; sprinkle with chocolate powder and you will have a soap which looks like a mocha!

Honey & Dandelion Soap

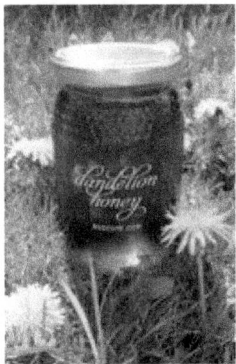

You can use dandelions to make your soap but this may result in bits in your soap! It is better to make a dandelion tea and use this to flavor the soap. The ingredients you will need are are; 10 ounces of dandelion tea and one ounce of honey. These two ingredients need to be added base soap once you have melted it. You should keep the soap simmering to ensure the honey and dandelion tea has mixed completely.

Again, this soap should be set within a few hours; ideally it should be used within three months of its first use.

Cucumber soap

Cucumber is known to clean and refresh any skin, adding it to a soap means you have access to it whenever you need a boost.

To make the soap you will need the pulp of one cucumber. The best way of doing this is to peel and grate it into the smallest pieces possible. Again, you will need to add this to the soap base and warm the entire mixture. It should be set within a few hours.

Soap on a stick

This can be a great way to introduce children to soap and remind everyone of how important it is to wash. Putting soap on a stick may make it appear like a lollipop; you will need to be careful that your children do not try to eat them!

You will need lollipop sticks; clear glycerin, food coloring and fragrance oil. Simply start by cutting the glycerin into blocks and putting them in a bowl before melting them in the microwave. You can then stir in your fragrance, the food coloring and any specific flavor your children may want to wash in. The mixture can then be poured into a mold and a lollipop stick attached. To get the soap to set it is best to put the molds in the freezer for ten minutes.

Conclusion

Making soap is cost effective, fun and will allow you to be extremely creative. There are literally hundreds of recipes, some will use lye whilst others use old soaps or soap base. It can often be good to start with the soap bases and move up to using lye mixtures. This will ensure you are comfortable with all the processes and measuring before tackling the more dangerous approach.

Providing you adopt a cautious approach to lye and always have a bottle of vinegar on standby you will be perfectly safe and capable of using lye. It does give off noxious fumes when first mixed, if possible it is better to mix it outside. However, providing you adopt the right approach you will not have an issue using this product.

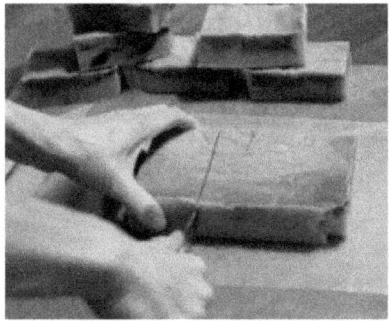

It is also fascinating to note how the scent and even the feel of soap can be completely changed just by increasing or decreasing the quantities of the ingredients. There is no reason why you cannot adjust the quantities or even add extra items to any recipe to make your own variant of soap; at the worst it will not work properly and you can simply start again!

Making your own soap is becoming increasingly popular; this is not just because it is much cheaper than buying luxury soap; there is also a sense of satisfaction and achievement when you make your first batch. In fact, it is so easy to get started in that there is really no excuse for anyone not to have a go!

FREE Bonus Reminder

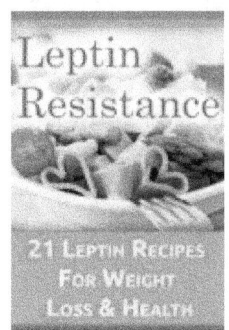

If you have not grabbed it yet, please go ahead and download your special bonus report *"Leptin Resistance. 21 Leptin Recipes For Weight Loss & Healthy Living"*.

Simply Click the Button Below

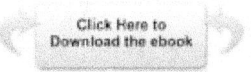

OR **Go to This Page**

http://easyweightlossway.com/free/

BONUS #2: More Free & Discounted Books

Do you want to receive more Free & Discounted Books?

We have a mailing list where we send out our new Books when they go free or with a discount on Kindle. Click on the link below to sign up for Free & Discount Book Promotions.

=> Sign Up for Free & Discount Book Promotions <=

OR Go to this URL

http://zbit.ly/1WBb1Ek